50 Easy-to-Prepare Air Fryer Recipes
The Ultimate Guide to Prepare Delicious and Healthier Food with Your Air Fryer

By
Elena Brown

In no way is it legal to reproduce, duplicate, or transmit any part of this document in either electronic means or in printed format. Recording of this publication is strictly prohibited, and any storage of this document is not allowed unless with written permission from the publisher. All rights reserved.

The information provided herein is stated to be truthful and consistent, in that any liability, in terms of inattention or otherwise, by any usage or abuse of any policies, processes, or directions contained within is the solitary and utter responsibility of the recipient reader. Under no circumstances will any legal responsibility or blame be

3

4

owned by the owners themselves, not affiliated with this document.

Table of Contents

Introduction

Magic it seems, technology it is: for some time now, we can find in the market fryers that work without bathing the food in hot oil. The responsible for this paradox is the hot air, which circulating at high temperature and certain speed cooks the food in a way quite similar to oil, but without that large amount of added fat. Although we will have to add a little if we want to get the characteristic golden and crispy crust, the difference in the lightness of one system and the other is abysmal.

But, in addition to making potatoes, croquettes, and breaded pork loin, air fryers offer a lot of culinary possibilities.

5 Tips for Better Air Frying

1. **Dry food thoroughly.** Before air frying, dry anything (without breading) that you want crispy or browned,

such as meat, fish, and vegetables.

2. **Avoid overfilling the basket.** An air fryer relies on a fan to circulate hot air and cook food quickly. If you overfill the basket, this prevents the hot air from reaching all the food, which slows cooking and can give uneven, mushy results. Some models have lines for maximum fill, and the manual may also provide instructions. As a general rule, our experts say not to fill the basket more than 3/4 parts if the basket does not have a maximum fill line.

3. **Check the food frequently.** Unlike cooking food in the oven, you can't turn on the light and check food cooking through the window. With an air fryer, you can't see the ingredients as they cook-they're placed in a drawer-style basket, which makes it harder to get a sense of how

it's going. And our staff found that cooking times can vary considerably. To avoid overcooked food, check it from time to time as it cooks. (On some models, this is as simple as pulling out the drawer, but on others, you may need to stop cooking before doing so; your manual will have specific information).

4. **Turn the food while cooking.** Use tongs or shake the basket during cooking for more even results.

5. **Experiment with home favorites.** Sure, store-bought fries taste great, but an air fryer makes the job easier: For crispy homemade fries, cut potatoes into uniform chunks and soak them in water for 30 minutes. Then drain, rinse, dry, and coat lightly with oil before air frying.

Keep in mind that temperatures and cooking times will vary depending on the fryer you use.

Chapter 1. Breakfast Recipes

In this chapter, we have compiled amazing and wholesome AirFryer breakfast recipes.

1. Tasty Baked Eggs

(Ready in about 20 mins | Serving 4 | Easy)

Ingredients:

- Four eggs
- One-pound of torn baby spinach
- Seven ounces of chopped ham
- Four tablespoons of milk
- One tablespoon of olive oil
- Cooking spray
- Salt and black pepper to the taste

Directions:

1. Prepare a pan of oil over medium pressure, add baby spinach, cook, and simmer for a few minutes.

2. Grate 4 spray ramekins and break the baby spinach and ham in each of them.
3. Season with salt and pepper. Put ramekins on preheated AirFryer at 350° F and bread in each ramekin for twenty minutes.
4. Baked eggs are ready to be served in breakfast.
5. Enjoy!

Nutrition: Calories: 321, Fat: 6g, Fiber: 8g, Carbs: 15g, Protein: 12g.

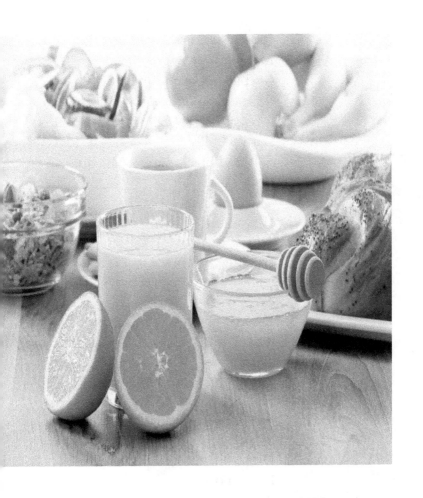

2. Breakfast Egg Bowls

(Ready in about 20 mins | Serving 4 | Easy)

Ingredients:

- 4 dinner rolls, chopped the tops off and scooped out the insides
- 4 tablespoons of hot cream
- Four chickens
- 4 teaspoons of chives mixed with parsley
- Salt and black pepper as you prefer
- 4 teaspoons of brushed Parmesan

Instructions:

3. Arrange dinner rolls and smash every egg on a bakery tray.
4. Divide heavy cream, mixed herbs, and salt through the season.
5. Sprinkle your rolls with parmesan, put it in your air bowl and cook for 20 minutes at 350° F.
6. Divide between plates the bread bowls.

7. Enjoy!

Nutrition: Calories: 238, Fat: 4g,
Fiber: 7g, Carbs: 14g, Protein: 7g.

3. Delicious Breakfast Soufflé

(Ready in about 16 mins | Serving 2 | Easy)

Ingredients:

- 4 eggs, whisked
- 4 tablespoons of heavy cream
- A pinch of red chili pepper, crushed
- 2 tablespoons of parsley, chopped
- 2 tablespoons of chives, chopped
- Salt and black pepper to the taste

Directions:

1. Mix the eggs with salt, pepper, heavy cream, red chili pepper, parsley, chives in a pot, stir well, and split into 4 dishes of soufflé.
2. Arrange dishes in the AirFryer and cook the soufflés for 8 minutes at 350° F.
3. Serve them.
4. Enjoy!

Nutrition: Calories: 300, Fat: 7g, Fiber: 9g, Carbs: 15g, Protein: 6g.

4. Air Fried Sandwich

(Ready in about 16 mins | Serving 2 | Easy)

Ingredients:

- 2 English muffins halved
- 2 eggs
- 2 bacon strips
- Salt and black pepper to the taste

Directions:

1. Crack eggs in your AirFryer, put bacon on top, cover, and cook at 392° F for 6 minutes.
2. Warm up the English muffin halves in the microwave for a few seconds, split eggs into two halves, place bacon on top, sprinkle salt and pepper, cover with the other two English muffins and serve for breakfast.
3. Enjoy!

Nutrition: Calories: 261, Fat: 5g, Fiber: 8g, Carbs: 12g, Protein: 4g.

5. Rustic Breakfast

(Ready in about 16 mins | Serving 2 | Easy)

Ingredients:

- 7 ounces baby spinach
- 8 chestnuts mushrooms, halved
- 8 tomatoes, halved
- 1 garlic clove, minced
- 4 chipolatas
- 4 bacon slices, chopped
- Salt and black pepper to the taste
- 4 eggs
- Cooking spray

Directions:

1. Grease the oil over a frying pan and add onions, garlic, and mushrooms.

2. Add bacon and chipolatas, and finish with spinach and crack eggs.

3. Cover with salt and pepper, bring the pan into your AirFryer's cooking basket, and cook at 350° F for 13 minutes.

4. Serve for breakfast.

5. Enjoy!

Nutrition: Calories: 312, Fat: 6g, Fiber: 8g, Carbs: 15g, Protein: 5g.

Chapter 2. Sides, Snacks and Appetizers Recipes

6. Prosciutto-Wrapped Parmesan Asparagus

(Ready in about 20 min | Servings 4 | Normal)

Ingredients:

- 1-pound of asparagus
- 12 (0.5-ounce) slices of prosciutto
- 1 tablespoon of coconut oil, melted
- 2 teaspoons of lemon juice
- 1/8 teaspoon of red pepper flakes
- 1/3 cup of grated Parmesan cheese
- 2 tablespoons of salted butter, melted

Directions:

1. Place an asparagus spear onto a slice of prosciutto on a clean work surface.

2. Drizzle with the lemon juice and coconut oil. Sprinkle over asparagus with red pepper flakes and Parmesan. Roll prosciutto with a spear of asparagus. Put the basket into the AirFryer.
3. Set the temperature to 375° F and set the timer for a further 10 minutes.
4. Before eating, sprinkle asparagus roll with butter.
5. Enjoy!

Nutrition: Calories: 263, Protein: 13.9g Fiber: 2.4g, Net Carbohydrates: 4.3g, Fat: 20.2g, Sodium: 368 mg, Carbohydrates: 6.7g, Sugar: 2.2g

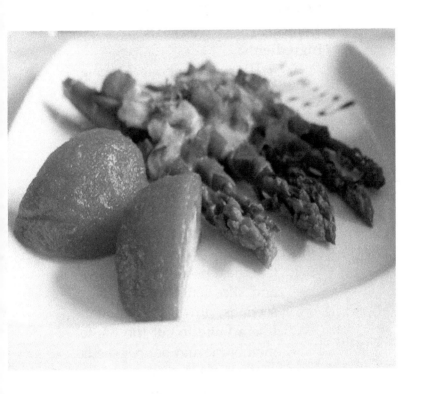

7. Bacon-Wrapped Jalapeño Poppers

(Ready in about 27 min | Servings 4 | Normal)

Ingredients:

- 6 jalapeños (about 4" long each)
- 3-ounces of full-Fat: cream cheese
- 1/3 cup of shredded medium Cheddar cheese
- 1/4 teaspoon of garlic powder
- 12 slices sugar-free bacon

Directions:

1. Cut the tops off the jalapeños and slice lengthwise in two sections down the middle. Use a knife to cut the white membrane and pepper seeds with caution.

2. Place the cream cheese, Cheddar, and garlic powder in a large microwave-safe dish. Microwave, then stir for 30 seconds. Mixture the spoon of cheese with the jalapeños.

26

3. Wrap a strip of bacon around half of each jalapeño, shielding the pepper entirely. Put the basket into the AirFryer.
4. Set the temperature to 400° F and change the timer for 12 minutes.
5. Switch the peppers halfway through the cycle of preparation. Serve warm.

Nutrition: Calories: 246, Protein: 14.4g, Fiber: 0.6g, Net Carbohydrates: 2.0g Fat: 17.9g, Sodium: 625 mg, Carbohydrates: 2.6g sugar: 1.6g.

8. Garlic Parmesan Chicken Wings

(Ready in about 30 min | Servings 4 | Normal)

Ingredients:

- 2 pounds of raw chicken wings
- 1 teaspoon of pink Himalayan salt
- 1/2 teaspoon of garlic powder
- 1 tablespoon of baking powder
- 4 tablespoons of unsalted butter, melted
- 1/3 cup of grated Parmesan cheese
- 1/4 teaspoon of dried parsley

Directions:

1. In a large bowl, place chicken wings, salt, ½ teaspoon of garlic powder, baking powder, and then toss. Place wings into the AirFryer basket.

2. Adjust the temperature to 400°F and set the timer for 25 minutes.
3. Toss the basket two or three times during the cooking time.
4. In a small bowl, combine butter, parmesan, and parsley.
5. Remove wings from the fryer and place it into a large clean bowl. Pour the butter mixture over the wings and toss until coated. Serve warm.
6. Enjoy!

Nutrition: Calories: 565, Protein: 41.8g, Fiber: 0.1g, Net Carbohydrates: 2.1g Fat: 42.g, Sodium: 1,067 mg, Carbohydrates: 2.2g sugar: 0.0g.

9. Spicy Buffalo Chicken Dip

(Ready in about 20 min | Servings 4 | Easy)

Ingredients:

- 1 cup of cooked, diced chicken breast
- 8 ounces of full-Fat: cream cheese, softened
- 1/2 cup of buffalo sauce
- 1/3 cup of full-Fat: ranch dressing
- 1/3 cup of chopped pickled jalapeños
- 1 ½ cups of shredded medium Cheddar cheese, divided
- 2 scallions, sliced

Directions:

1. Place chicken into a large bowl. Add cream cheese, buffalo sauce, and ranch dressing. Stir until the spices are well mixed and mostly smooth. Fold in jalapeños and 1 cup Cheddar.
2. Pour the mixture into a 4-cup round baking dish and place

the remaining Cheddar on top. Place the dish into the AirFryer basket.

3. Adjust the temperature to 350°F and set the timer for 10 minutes.

4. When done, the top will be brown and bubbling. Top with sliced scallions. Serve warm.

5. Enjoy!

Nutrition: Calories: 472 Protein: 25.6g, Fiber: 0.6g, Net Carbohydrates: 8.5g Fat: 32.0g, Sodium: 1,532 mg, Carbohydrates: 9.1g sugar: 7.4g.

10. Bacon Jalapeño Cheese Bread

(Ready in about 25 min | Servings 2 | Yields 8 sticks (2 sticks per serving) | Normal)

Ingredients:

- 2 cups of shredded mozzarella cheese
- ¼ cup of grated Parmesan cheese
- ¼ cup of chopped pickled jalapeños
- 2 large eggs
- 4 slices of sugar-free bacon, cooked and chopped

Directions:

1. Mix all ingredients in a large bowl. Cut a piece of parchment to fit your AirFryer basket.
2. Dampen your hands with a bit of water and press out the mixture into a circle. You may need to separate this into two smaller cheese bread, depending on your fryer's size.

3. Place the parchment and cheese bread into the AirFryer basket.
4. Adjust the temperature to 320°F and set the timer for 15 minutes.
5. Carefully flip the bread when 5 minutes remain.
6. When fully cooked, the top will be golden brown. Serve warm and enjoy!

Nutrition: Calories: 273, Protein: 20.1g, Fiber: 0.1g, Net Carbohydrates: 2.1g Fat: 18.1g, Sodium: 749 mg, Carbohydrates: 2.3g, sugar: 0.7g.

11.Pizza Rolls

(Ready in about 25 min | Servings 3
| Yields 24 rolls (3 per serving) |
Normal)

Ingredients:

- 2 cups of shredded mozzarella cheese
- 1/2 cup of almond flour 2 large eggs
- 72 slices of pepperoni
- 8 (1-ounce) mozzarella string cheese sticks, cut into 3 pieces
- 2 tablespoons of unsalted butter, melted
- 1/4 teaspoon of garlic powder
- ½ teaspoon of dried parsley
- 2 tablespoons of grated Parmesan cheese

Directions:

1. In a large microwave-safe bowl, place mozzarella and almond flour. Microwave for 1 minute. Remove bowl and mix until forming a ball of dough. Microwave

additional 30 seconds if necessary.

2. Crack eggs into the bowl and mix until smooth dough ball forms. Wet your hands with water and knead the dough briefly.

3. Tear off two large pieces of parchment paper and spray one side of each with non-stick cooking spray.

4. Place the dough ball between the two sheets, with sprayed sides facing dough. Use a rolling pin to roll the dough out to ¼ " thickness.

5. Use a knife to slice into 24 rectangles. On each rectangle, place 3 pepperoni slices and 1-piece string cheese.

6. Fold the rectangle in half, covering pepperoni and cheese filling. Pinch or roll sides closed. Cut a piece of parchment to fit your AirFryer basket and place it into the basket. Put the rolls onto the parchment.

7. Adjust the temperature to 350°F and set the timer for 10 minutes.
8. After 5 minutes, open the fryer and flip the pizza rolls. Restart the fryer and continue cooking until pizza rolls are golden.
9. In a small bowl, place butter, garlic powder, and parsley. Brush the mixture over cooked pizza rolls and then sprinkle with Parmesan. Serve warm.

Nutrition: Calories: 333, Protein: 20.7g, Fiber: 0.8g, Net Carbohydrates: 2.5g Fat: 24.0g, Sodium: 708 mg, Carbohydrates: 3.3g, Sugar: 0.9g.

12. Bacon Cheeseburger Dip

(Ready in about 30 min | Servings 6 | Normal)

Ingredients:

- 8 ounces of full-Fat: cream cheese
- 1/4 cup of full-Fat: mayonnaise
- 1/4 cup of full-Fat: sour cream
- 1/4 cup of chopped onion
- 1 teaspoon of garlic powder
- 1 tablespoon of Worcestershire sauce 1
- 1/4 cups of shredded medium Cheddar cheese, divided
- ½-pound of cooked 80/20 ground beef
- 6 slices of sugar-free bacon, cooked and crumbled
- 2 large of pickle spears, chopped.

Directions:

1. In a large microwave-safe bowl, place the cream cheese and microwave for 45

seconds. Stir in mayonnaise, sour cream, onion, powdered garlic, and one cup of Worcestershire Cheddar sauce. Add the bacon and the ground beef. Sprinkle over leftover Cheddar.

2. Place the bowl in 6 "and put it in the basket of the AirFryer.
3. Set the temperature to 400° F and adjust the timer for 10 minutes.
4. When the top is golden, bubbling sprinkles the pickles over the dish and serves warm.

Nutrition: Calories: 457, Protein: 21.6g, Fiber: 0.2g, Net Carbohydrates: 3.6g Fat: 35.0g, Sodium: 589 mg, Carbohydrates: 3.8g, Sugar: 2.2g.

13. Pork Rind Tortillas

(Ready in about 15 min | Servings 4
| Yields 4 tortillas (1 per serving) |
Easy)

Ingredients:

- 1-ounce of pork rinds
- 3/4 cup of shredded mozzarella cheese
- 2 tablespoons of full-Fat: cream cheese
- 1 large egg

Directions:

1. Install pork rinds in a food processor and pulse until finely soiled.
2. Place the mozzarella in a large, safe microwave bowl. Break-in small pieces of the cream cheese and add to the bowl. Microwave for 30 seconds, or until both kinds of cheese are melted and easily stirred into a ball. To the cheese mixture, add the ground pork rinds and the egg.
3. Continue to stir till the mixture forms a ball. If it

cools too much and hardens the cheese, then microwave for another 10 seconds.

4. Set the dough aside into four small balls. Place each dough ball between two parchment sheets, and roll into a 1/4 flat layer.

5. Place tortillas in a single layer AirFryer basket; work in batches where necessary.

6. Set the temperature to 400° F and adjust the timer for 5 minutes.

7. When fully cooked, the tortillas will become crispy and firm. Serve immediately and enjoy!

Nutrition: Calories: 145, Protein: 10.7g, Fiber: 0.0g, Net Carbohydrates: 0.8g Fat: 10.0g, Sodium: 291 mg, Carbohydrates: 0.8g, Sugar: 0.5g.

14. Mozzarella Sticks

(Ready in about 1 hour 10 min | Servings 3 | Yields 12 sticks (3 per serving) | Normal)

Ingredients:

- 6 (1-ounce) mozzarella string cheese sticks
- 1/2 cup of grated Parmesan cheese
- ½- an ounce of pork rinds, finely ground
- 1 teaspoon of dried parsley
- 2 large eggs

Directions:

15. Put the sticks of mozzarella on a cutting board and cut in half. Freeze to stand for 45 minutes or until solid. When freezing overnight, cut frozen sticks after 1 hour and put them in an airtight zip-top storage bag for future use.

16. Combine the Parmesan, ground pork rinds, and parsley in a large bowl.

17. Then whisk eggs in a medium bowl.

18. Brush a frozen mozzarella over beaten eggs, then coat in a Parmesan sauce. Repeat for unused sticks. Place the mozzarella sticks in the bowl of the AirFryer.
19. Adjust the temperature to 400° F and set the timer to golden for 10 minutes.
20. Serve hot and enjoy!

Nutrition: Calories: 236, Protein: 19.2g Fiber: 0.0g, Net Carbohydrates: 4.7g Fat: 13.8g, Sodium: 609 mg Carbohydrates: 4.7g, Sugar: 1.1g.

15. Bacon-Wrapped Onion Rings

(Ready in about 15 min | Servings 4 | Normal)

Ingredients:

- 1 large onion, peeled
- 1 tablespoon of sriracha
- 8 slices of sugar-free bacon

Directions:

1. Slice of the ointment into 1/4"-thick slices. Take two slices of onion and tie the bacon around the rings. Repeat for the remaining onion and bacon.
2. Set the temperature to 350° F and change the timer for 10 minutes.
3. Use pliers to rotate the onion rings halfway through the cooking time. Bacon will be crispy when fully fried. Eat hot and enjoy it!

Nutrition: Calories: 105, Protein: 7.5 g Fiber: 0.6g Net Carbohydrates: 3.7g Fat: 5.9g, Sodium: 401 mg Carbohydrates: 4.3g sugar: 2.3g.

Chapter 3.
Vegetable and Vegetarian Recipes

16.Masala Galette

(Ready in about 15 min | Servings 2 | Easy)

Ingredients:

- 2 tbsp. of garam masala
- 2 medium potatoes boiled and mashed
- 1 ½ cup of coarsely crushed peanuts
- 3 tsp. of ginger finely chopped
- 1-2 tbsp. of fresh coriander leaves
- 2 or 3 green chilies finely chopped
- 1 ½ tbsp. of lemon juice
- Salt and pepper to taste

Directions:

1. Blend the ingredients into a sterile tub.
2. Form this mixture into flat and circular galettes.

3. Wet the galettes with water gently. Cover with smashed peanuts on each galette.
4. Preheat the AirFryer for 5 minutes, at 160° Fahrenheit. Place your
5. Fry basket galettes and let them steam for another 25 minutes at the bottom
6. Just at the same temperature. Go turning them over to get to fry. Serve with ketchup or mint chutney.

Nutrition: Calories: 250 kcal.

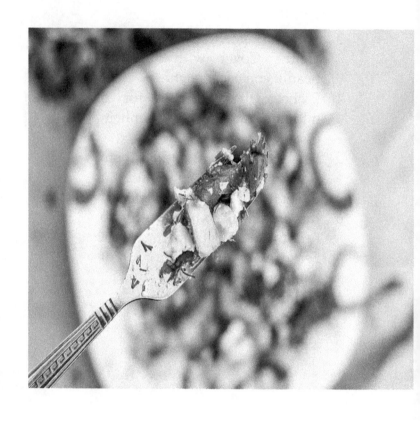

17.Potato Samosa

(Ready in about 30 min | Servings 6 | Normal)

Ingredients:

For wrappers:

- 2 tbsp. of unsalted butter
- 1 ½ cup of all-purpose flour
- A pinch of salt to taste
- Add as much water as required to make the dough stiff and firm

For filling:

- 2-3 big potatoes boiled and mashed
- ¼ cup of boiled peas
- 1 tsp. of powdered ginger
- 1 or 2 green chilies that are finely chopped or mashed
- ½ tsp. of cumin
- 1 tsp. of coarsely crushed coriander
- 1 dry red chili broken into pieces
- A small amount of salt (to the taste)
- ½ tsp. of dried mango powder
- ½ tsp. of red chili powder.

- 1-2 tbsp. of coriander.

Directions:

1. Rub the dough to make it rigid to flat for exterior wrapping. Let it rest in a jar until the filling is finished.

2. Heat the ingredients in a saucepan and mix well to create a sticky paste. Print out the bread.

3. Wrap the dough into balls and flatten. Break them in half and then apply the filling. Use water to help you fold the rims and make a cone shape.

4. Preheat the AirFryer at 300 Fahrenheit for around 5-6 minutes. In the fry basket, put all the samosas and close the basket properly. Hold the AirFryer for another 20 to 25 minutes, at 200°.

5. Open the basket at the halfway mark, and turn over the samosas for standard preparation. After this, fry for around 10 minutes at 250° to give them the perfect

golden-brown hue. Serve wet. Recommended sides are chutney with tamarind or mint.

Nutrition: Calories: 150 kcal.

18. Vegetable Kebab

(Ready in about 30 min | Servings 2 | Normal)

Ingredients:

- 2 cups of mixed vegetables
- 3 onions chopped
- 5 green chilies-roughly chopped
- 1 ½ tbsp. of ginger paste
- 1 ½ tsp. of garlic paste
- 1 ½ tsp. of salt
- 3 tsp. of lemon juice
- 2 tsp. of garam masala
- 4 tbsp. of chopped coriander
- 3 tbsp. of cream
- 3 tbsp. of chopped capsicum
- 3 eggs
- 2 ½ tbsp. of white sesame seeds

Directions:

1. Except for the egg, grind the ingredients, and create a smooth paste. Coat the cover paste foods. Beat the eggs now, and apply more salt to it.
2. In the egg mixture, scatter the coated vegetables and move

to the sesame seeds and garnish well with herbs. Place the vegetables onto a stick.

3. Pre fire up the AirFryer for about 5 minutes at 160° Fahrenheit. Place sticks in the basket and cook for another 25 minutes

4. Just at the same temperature, switch the clamps during the cooking process to the cook's suit.

Nutrition: Calories: 115 kcal.

19.Sago Galette

(Ready in about 25 min | Servings 2 | Normal)

Ingredients:

- 2 cups of sago soaked
- 1 ½ cup of coarsely crushed peanuts
- 3 tsp. of ginger finely chopped
- 1-2 tbsp. of fresh coriander leaves
- 2 or 3 green chilies finely chopped
- 1 ½ tbsp. of lemon juice
- Salt and pepper to the taste

Directions:

1. Wash the soaked sago, then put it in a clean bowl with the other ingredients. Form this mixture into flat and circular galettes.
2. Wet the galettes with water gently. Cover with smashed peanuts on each galette.
3. Preheat the AirFryer for 5 minutes, at 160° Fahrenheit. Place your fry basket galettes and let them steam for

another 25 minutes at the bottom just the same temperature. Go turning them over to get to fry. Serve with chutney, basil, or ketchup.

Nutrition: Calories: 220 kcal.

20. Stuffed Capsicum Baskets

(Ready in about 25 min | Servings 2 | Normal)

Ingredients:

<u>For baskets:</u>

- 3-4 long capsicum
- ½ tsp. of salt
- ½ tsp. of pepper powder

<u>For filling:</u>

- 1 medium onion finely chopped
- 1 green chili finely chopped
- 2 or 3 large potatoes boiled and mashed
- 1 ½ tbsp. of chopped coriander leaves
- 1 tsp. of fenugreek
- 1 tsp. of dried mango powder
- 1 tsp. of cumin powder
- Salt and pepper to the taste

<u>For topping:</u>

- 3 tbsp. of grated cheese
- 1 tsp. of red chili flakes
- ½ tsp. of oregano
- ½ tsp. of basil

- ½ tsp. of parsley

Directions:

1. Take all the ingredients and put them together in a tub under the heading "Filling."
2. Take off the capsicum stem. Break the caps off. Take off seeds as well.
3. Sprinkle some salt and pepper over the capsicum inside. Turn on until they've been apart for some time.
4. Now fill in the hollowed-out capsicums with the planned filling. Sprinkle the grated cheese, then apply the seasoning as well.
5. Preheat the AirFryer for 5 minutes at 140° Fahrenheit. Place the capsicums in and near the fry basket. Let them cook likewise 20 Minutes more temperature. Switch them in between to escape up cooking.

Nutrition: Calories: 235 kcal.

21. Baked Macaroni Pasta

(Ready in about 25 min | Servings 2 | Normal)

Ingredients:

- 1 cup of pasta
- 7 cups of boiling water
- 1 ½ tbsp. of olive oil
- A pinch of salt

For tossing pasta:

- 1 ½ tbsp. of olive oil
- ½ cup of small carrot pieces
- Salt and pepper to the taste
- ½ tsp. of oregano
- ½ tsp. of basil

For the white sauce:

- 2 tbsp. of olive oil
- 2 tbsp. of all-purpose flour
- 2 cups of milk
- 1 tsp. of dried oregano
- ½ tsp. of dried basil
- ½ tsp. of dried parsley
- Salt and pepper to the taste

Directions:

1. When done, cook the pasta and sieve. Toss the pasta in the above-mentioned ingredients and set aside.

Apply the ingredients to a skillet for the sauce, and bring them to a boil.

2. Drop the sauce and keep simmering to make a thicker sauce. Apply the pasta to the sauce and pass it into cheese-garnished glass dish.

3. Preheat the AirFryer for 5 minutes, at 160°. Place in the bowl basket, and fasten it. At the same temperature, let it continue to cook for 10 minutes. Hold stirring in the sauce.

Nutrition: Calories: 245 kcal.

22.Macaroni Samosa

(Ready in about 30 min | Servings 2 | Normal)

Ingredients:

<u>For wrappers:</u>

- 1 cup of all-purpose flour
- 2 tbsp. of unsalted butter
- A pinch of salt to the taste
- Take the amount of water sufficient enough to make a stiff dough

<u>For filling:</u>

- 3 cups of boiled macaroni
- 2 onion sliced
- 2 capsicum sliced
- 2 carrot sliced
- 2 cabbage sliced
- 2 tbsp. of soya sauce
- 2 tsp. of vinegar
- 2 tbsp. of ginger finely chopped
- 2 tbsp. of garlic finely chopped
- 2 tbsp. of green chilies finely chopped
- 2 tbsp. of ginger-garlic paste
- Some salt and pepper to taste
- 2 tbsp. of olive oil

- ½ tsp. of ajinomoto

Directions:

1. Rub the dough to make it rigid to flat for exterior wrapping. Set it aside rest in a tub while the filling is finished.

2. Heat the ingredients in a saucepan and mix well to create a sticky paste. Function out the paint.

3. Wrap the dough into balls and flatten. Break-in half, then add the filling up. Using water to help you fold the rims and make a cone shape.

4. Preheat the AirFryer at 300 Fahrenheit for about 5-6 minutes. Place everything in one place the fry basket samosas, then lock the basket properly. Hold the AirFryer for another 20 to 25 minutes, at 200°.

5. Open the bowl and turn the samosas over to cook evenly. Afterward, fry for about 10 minutes at 250°, to give them the desired hue of a golden tan.   Serve   wet.

Recommended sides contain
tamarinds or green chutney.
Nutrition: Calories: 230.

23.Burritos

(Ready in about 35 min | Servings 2 | Normal)

Ingredients:

Refried beans:

- ½ cup of red kidney beans (soaked overnight)
- ½ small onion chopped
- 1 tbsp. of olive oil
- 2 tbsp. of tomato puree
- ¼ tsp. of red chili powder
- 1 tsp. of salt to the taste
- 4-5 flour tortillas

Vegetable Filling:

- 1 tbsp. of olive oil
- 1 medium onion finely sliced
- 3 flakes of garlic crushed
- ½ cup of French beans (Slice them lengthwise into thin and long slices)
- ½ cup of mushrooms thinly sliced
- 1 cup of cottage cheese cut in too long and slightly thick fingers
- ½ cup of shredded cabbage
- 1 tbsp. of coriander, chopped
- 1 tbsp. of vinegar

- 1 tsp. of white wine
- A pinch of salt to the taste
- ½ tsp. of red chili flakes
- 1 tsp. of freshly ground peppercorns
- ½ cup of pickled jalapenos (Chop them up finely)
- 2 carrots (Cut into long thin slices)

Salad:

- 1-2 lettuce leaves shredded.
- 1 or 2 spring onions chopped finely. Also, cut the greens.
- 1 tomato. Remove the seeds and chop it into small pieces.
- 1 green chili chopped.
- 1 cup of cheddar cheese, grated.

Directions:

1. Cook the beans along with the onion and garlic and mash them finely. Now, make the sauce you will need for the burrito. Ensure that you create a slightly thick sauce.

2. For the filling, you will need to cook the ingredients well in a pan and ensure that the

vegetables have browned on the outside.

3. To make the salad, toss the ingredients together. Place the tortilla and add a sauce layer, followed by the beans and the filling at the center. Before you roll it, you will need to place the salad on top of the filling.

4. Preheat the AirFryer for around 5 minutes at 200 Fahrenheit. Open the fry basket and keep the burritos inside. Close the basket properly. Let the AirFryer remains at 200 Fahrenheit for another 15 minutes or so.

5. Halfway through, remove the basket and turn all the burritos over to get a uniform cook.

Nutrition: Calories: 275 kcal.

Chapter 4. Pork, Beef, and Lamb Recipes

24.Beef Roll

(Ready in about 24 min | Servings 4 | Normal)
Ingredients:
2 lbs. of steak beef, open and compressed with a meat mallet
Salt and black pepper, to satisfy
1 cup of spinach
3 ounces of red bell pepper, cooked and diced
Six Provolone Cheese Slices
Pesto: 3 Teaspoons
Directions:
1. Organize flat beef steak on a baking sheet, spray pesto all over the place. Place the cheese in one plate, place the chili peppers, spinach, and salt and potatoes to try.
2. Roll your burger, save on matchsticks, sprinkle with salt and then pepper, put the

roll in the basket of your AirFryer, and cook 400 F for 14 minutes, turning halfway around the roll.

3. Place aside to cool, cut into rolls 2 inches smaller. Serve as an appetizer.

Nutrition: Calories: 230, Fat: 1g, Carbohydrates 12g, Protein:

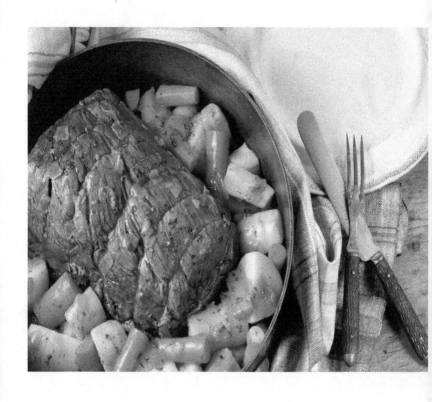

25.Empanada

(Ready in about 35 min | Servings 4 | Normal)

Ingredients:

- 1 box of shells of empanada
- 1 liter of olive oil
- 1 lb of beef, processed meat
- 1 yellow onion, sliced
- Salt and black chili, to satisfy
- 2 cloves of garlic, diced
- 1/2 cumin cubicle, land
- 1/4 cup of tomatoes salsa
- 1 whisked egg yolk and 1 tablespoon of water
- 1 green, chopped bell pepper

Directions:

1. Burn up a saucepan with the oil at low pressure, and add the beef.
2. Stir in onion, garlic, lime, chili pepper, bell pepper, and tomato salsa. Then pump it up for 15 minutes.
3. Split grilled beef into shells of empanada, sprinkle with beaten egg, and seal it off.

4. Put in the large pan of your AirFryer, and cook at 350 F for Ten minutes
5. Prepare on a tray, and serve as an appetizer.
6. Enjoy!

Nutrition: Calories:274, Fat: 17g, Fiber:14g, Carbohydrates 20g, Protein: 7g.

26.Pork Rolls

(Ready in about 50 min | Servings 4 | Normal)

Ingredients:

- 15 ounce of prime rib of pork
- 1/2 teaspoon of cayenne pepper
- 1/4 tsp of powdered of cinnamon
- One clove of garlic, diced
- Salt and black chili, to try
- 2 pounds of olive oil
- 1 1/2 tsp, ground cumin
- One red onion, sliced
- Three cubits of parsley, chopped

Directions:

1. Mix the cinnamon in a bowl with the garlic, salt, pepper, chili powder, oil. Pick cumin and parsley and mix well.
2. Place pork fillet on a cutting board and flatten with a meat tenderizer, and to flatten with a beef tenderizer.
3. Blend the onion over the bacon, roll close, slice into moderate rolls. Heat at 360 °F

in the hot oven AirFryer and cook for 35 Mins.

4. Put them up on a plate and use it as an appetizer.
5. Enjoy!

Nutrition: Calories: 304, Fat: 12g, Fiber:1g, Carbohydrates 15g, Protein: 23g.

27.Rolls Beef Party

(Ready in about 25 min | Servings 4 | Normal)

Ingredients:

- 14 ounces of beef
- 7 ounces of white wine
- 4 cutlets of meat
- salt and black chili, to satisfy
- 8 sage leaves
- 4 pieces of ham
- 1 tablespoon butter, molten

Directions:

1. Warm up a pan on the stove with stock, insert wine. Heat once decreased, remove heat and disperse in small containers
2. Sprinkle with salt and chili pepper, fill with sage and roll each in sliced ham.
3. Put the rolls in butter, drop them in the bucket of your AirFryer, and cook for fifteen min, at 400° F.
4. Place rolls on a large plate and eat with the sausage.
5. Enjoy!

Nutrition: Calories: 260, Fat: 12g,
Fiber: 1g, Carbs: 22g, Protein: 21g.

28.Patties Beef

(Ready in about 18 min | Servings 4 | Normal)

Ingredients:

- Fourteen ounces of beef, chopped
- Two tablespoons ham, sliced into pieces
- One leek, sliced
- Three spoonfuls of bread crumbs
- Salt and black chili, to try
- Nutmeg 1/2 tsp, ground

Directions:

1. Mix the beef in a bowl with the leek, salt, pepper, ham, crumbs, and Nutmeg, stir well, and make tiny patties from the mixture.
2. Put in the basket of your AirFryer, cook at 400° F for 8 min. Set aside on a platter for minutes and serve as an appetizer.
3. Enjoy!

Nutrition: Calories: 260, Fat: 12g, fruit 3, Carbohydrates 12g, Protein: 21g

29. Greek Meatballs for Lamb

(Ready in about 18 min | Servings 10 | Normal)

Ingredients:

- Four Ounces of lamb beef, diced
- Salt and black chili, to taste
- One Piece of toasted, crushed bread
- Two Spoons of feta cheese, shattering
- 1/2 cubit lemon peel, grated
- One spoonful of oregano, minced

Directions:

1. Integrate meat and bread crumbs, salt , pepper, feta in a dish,
2. Mix properly, peel the oregano and lemon, form Ten meatballs and put them in the fryer.
3. Heat for 8 minutes at 400 °F, place it on a serving plate and appetizer to eat.
4. Enjoy!

Nutrition: Calories: 234, Fat: 12g,
Fiber: 2g, Carbohydrates 20g,
Protein: 20g

Chapter 5. Fish and Sea Food

30.Yummy Pollock

(Ready in about 25 min | Servings 6 | Normal)

Ingredients:

- 1/2 cup of sour cream
- Four pollock fillets, barefoot
- Parmesan: 1/4 cup, rubbed
- 2 tablespoons of sugar, melted
- Salt and black chili, to the taste
- Kitchen spray

Directions:

1. Mix the sour cream in a dish of butter, parmesan, salt, and pepper and whisk fine.
2. Sprinkle fish with spray to fry and season with salt and pepper.
3. Place the sour cream mixture on each side of. Pollock fillet, arrange in hot oven 320° F AirFryer, then cook for 15 minutes.

4. Divide Pollock fillets into bowls, and serve with a delightful side salad.
5. Enjoy!

Nutrition: Calories: 300, Fat: 13, Fiber: 3g, Carbohydrates 14g, Protein: 44g.

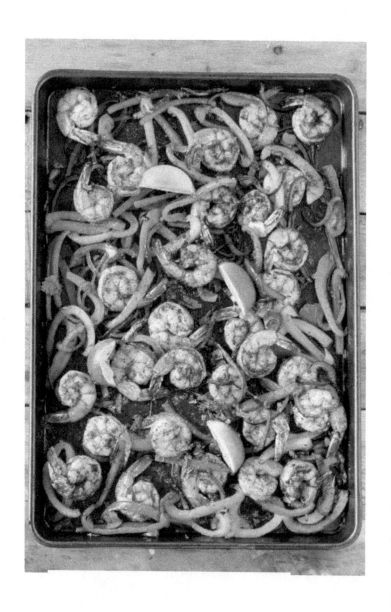

31.Honey Sea Bass

(Ready in about 20 min | Servings 2 | Normal)

Ingredients:

- 2 fillets of sea bass
- 1/2 orange zest, rubbed
- 1/2 fruit juice
- 1 tablespoon of black pepper and salt
- 2 mustard spoons
- 2 honey teaspoons
- 2 pounds of olive oil
- 1/2 pound of dried, drained lentils
- A tiny amount of dill, chopped
- 2 ounces of cress water
- A tiny amount of chopped parsley

Directions:

1. Add salt and peppered fish fillets, apply citrus zest and juice, rub with 1 spoonful of milk, honey and mustard, and pass to your air Fry and cook for 10 minutes at 350° F, turning in half.

2. In the meantime, place the lentils in a small pot, heat them up over medium heat, add them milk, watercress, dill and parsley, mix well and split between plates.
3. Insert the fish fillets and serve promptly.
4. Enjoy it!

Nutrition: Calories: 212, Fat: 8g, Fiber: 12g, Carbohydrates 9g, Protein: 17g.

32.Tilapia Sauce and Chives

(Ready in about 18 min | Servings 4 | Normal)

Ingredients:

- 4 Medium fillets with tilapia
- Cooking spray
- Salt and black chili, to satisfy
- 2 honey teaspoons
- Greek yogurt: 1⁄4 cup
- 1 lemon juice
- 2 spoonful of chives, chopped

Directions:

1. Season with salt and pepper, sprinkle with mist, put in hot oven 350° F AirFryer and cook for ten minutes, tossing midway.
2. In the meantime, blend yogurt with sugar, salt, vinegar, vinegar, and chives in a cup, whisk lemon juice.
3. Divide AirFryer fish into bowls, chop yogurt sauce and serve immediately.
4. Enjoy!

Nutrition: Calories: 261, Fat: 8g, Fiber: 18g, Carbohydrates 24g, Protein: 21g.

33. Tilapia Coconut

(Ready in about 20 min | Servings 4 | Normal)

Ingredients:

- 4 Medium fillets with tilapia
- Salt and black chili, to try
- 1/2 cup of cocoon milk
- 1 ginger-spoon, rubbed
- 1/2 cup of cilantro
- 2 sliced cloves of garlic
- 1/2 teaspoon of masala garam
- Cooking spray
- Half jalapeno, split

Directions:

1. Mix the coconut milk with salt, pepper, cilantro in your food processor, ginger, garlic, jalapeno, which masala garam, and always pulse well.

2. Sprinkle fish with cooking oil, scatter coconut mixes around, rub well. Switch to the basket with the AirFryer and cook at 400° F for 10 minutes.

3. Divide between plates and serve hot.

4. Enjoy!

Nutrition: Calories: 200, Fat: 5g, Fiber: 6g, Carbohydrates 25g, Protein: 26g.

34.Catfish Fillets Special

(Ready in about 22 min | Servings 4 | Normal)

Ingredients:

- 2 catfish fillets
- 1/2 teaspoon of ginger
- 2 ounces of butter
- 4 ounces of Worcestershire sauce
- 1/2 cubicle jerk seasoning
- 1 mustard casserole
- 1 spoonful of balsamic vinegar
- Catsup: 3/4 cup
- Salt and black chili, to try
- 1 spoonful of parsley, chopped

Directions:

1. Heat a skillet over medium heat with the butter, add Worcestershire seasoning of sauce, garlic, mustard, catsup, vinegar, salt, and hot pepper. Adjust fire, swirl well, and apply fish fillets.

2. Toss well, leave the fillets for 10 minutes, drain them, pass

them to the preheated oven, 350° F AirFryer basket and cook for 8 minutes halfway through flip fillets.

3. Divide into bowls, brush on top with parsley and serve immediately.

4. Enjoy!

Nutrition: Calories: 351, Fat: 8g, Fiber: 16g, Carbohydrates 27g, Protein: 17g.

Chapter 6. Poultry Recipes

35. Coconut Fluffy Chicken

(Ready in about 2hr 25 min | Servings 4 | Normal)

Ingredients:

- 4 large chicken legs
- Five spoons of turmeric powder
- Two ginger spoons, ground in
- Salt and black chili, to try
- Four tsp of coconut cream

Directions:

1. Comb the cream and the turmeric, ginger, salt, and pepper in a cup. Insert bits of chicken, toss well, and keep on for 2 hours.
2. Switch the chicken to your AirFryer and cook at 370° F. Divide into plates for 25 minutes, then serve with a side salad.
3. Enjoy!

Nutrition: Calories: 300, Fat: 4g, Fiber: 12g, Carbohydrates 22g, Protein: 20g.

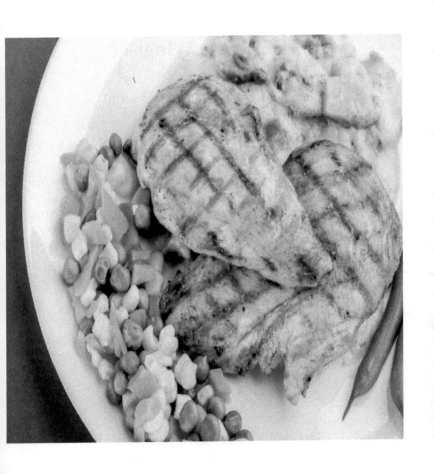

36. Chinese Wings of Chicken

(Ready in about 2hr 15 min | Servings 6 | Normal)

Ingredients:

- Sixteen wings of chicken
- 1 tbsp of honey
- 1 tbsp of soy sauce
- Salt and black chili, to try
- 1/4 tsp of white pepper
- Three spoonsful of lime juice

Directions:

1. Comb the honey and the soy sauce, salt, black and white pepper in a cup, and lime juice, shake well, add pieces of chicken and mix to cover. Hold in the refrigerator for 2 hours.

2. Switch the chicken to your AirFryer and cook for 6 at 370 °F for 6 Minutes, heat to 400° F, and cook for three minutes.

3. Serve wet and enjoy.

Nutrition: Calories: 372, Fat: 9g, Fiber: 10g, Carbohydrates 37g, Protein: 24g.

37.Chicken and Radish Mix

(Ready in about 40 min | Servings 4 | Normal)

Ingredients:

- Four stuffed chicken, bone-in
- Salt and black chili, to satisfy
- 1 tablespoon of olive oil
- 1 cup stock of chicken
- Six radishes, half cut
- 1 tsp of sugar
- Three carrots, thinly sliced into sticks
- Two spoonsful of chives, chopped

Directions:

1. Spontaneously ignite a saucepan that suits your fryer at medium pressure, add the stock, minimize heat to mild, carrots, sugar, and radishes. Stir gently, and partially cover the pot and cook for 20 minutes.

2. Rub the chicken with the oil, sprinkle with the salt and the pepper, bring in the olive oil

AirFryer, and cook for four minutes at 350° Fahrenheit.

3. Transfer the chicken to the radish mixture, toss and put all in the AirFryer, cook for another four minutes, split and start serving in plates.

4. Enjoy!

Nutrition: Calories: 237, Fat: 10g, Fiber: 4g, Carbohydrates 19g, Protein: 29g.

38.Glazed Chicken Tea

(Ready in about 40 min | Servings 6 | Normal)

Ingredients:

- 1/2 cup of apricot
- 1/2 cup of pineapple
- 6 chicken legs
- 1 cup of warm water
- Six functions of black tea
- 1 pound of soy sauce
- 1 onion, sliced
- 1/4 teaspoon of red chili flakes
- 1 tablespoon of olive oil
- Salt and black chili, to try

Directions:

1. Put the warm water in a bowl, add the tea bags, and leave to cover for discard bags at the end for 10 minutes and switch tea to another bowl.

2. Add soy sauce, pepper flakes, apricot preserves, and pineapples. Whisk thoroughly and heat off.

3. Season the chicken with salt and pepper, season with oil,

place in the AirFryer, and cook for 5 minutes, at 350° F.

4. Fanned onion on the lower part of an AirFryer-fitting baking dish, insert pieces of chicken, sprinkle the tea glaze on top, put in your AirFryer, and cook 25 minutes at 320° F.

5. On plates, divide everything and serve.

6. Enjoy!

Nutrition: Calories: 298, Fat:s 14g, Fiber: 1g, Carbs: 14g, Protein: 30g.

39.Chicken with Peaches

(Ready in about 40 min | Servings 4 | Normal)

Ingredients:

- Chicken in whole, sliced into moderate portions
- 3⁄4 cups of water
- 1/3 cups of honey
- Salt and black chili, to satisfy
- Olive oil: 1⁄4 cup
- 4 peaches, half

Directions:

1. Put the water in a kettle, bring over moderate heat to a boil, whisk very good and set it aside.

2. Rub the pieces of chicken with the grease, season with salt and pepper, and put in a bowl in your AirFryer at 350° F for ten min.

3. Put some of the honey mixtures in the chicken and cook for 6 minutes. Flip back, brush with the honey mix once more, and cook about 7 minutes.

4. Split pieces of chicken over plates and keep warm.
5. Place the peaches with what is left of the honey marinade. Fry them in the air and simmer for 3 minutes.
6. Divide around plates and serve next to pieces of chicken.
7. Enjoy!

Nutrition: Calories: 430, Fat: 14g, Carbohydrates 3g, sugars 15g, Protein: 20g.

40.Fast Fluffy Casserole Chicken

(Ready in about 22 min | Servings 4 | Normal)

Ingredients:

- 10 ounces of spinach, chopped
- Four cups of butter
- Three tablespoons of flour
- 1 and a half cups of milk
- 1/2 parmesan cup, ripened
- 1/2 cup of milk, hard
- Salt and black chili, to try
- Two cups of chicken breasts, skinless, ossified and cubed
- 1 cup of diced bread

Directions:

1. Burn up a pan over medium heat with butter, add the flour and mix well.
2. Stir well, simmer for 1-2 minutes, add milk, whipping cream and add parmesan to keep the pressure off.
3. Place chicken and spinach in a saucepan that suits your AirFryer.

4. Stir in salt and pepper, then toss.
5. Apply cream mixture and scatter, sprinkle the crumbs of bread over the end, place in the freezer the air and simmer for 12 minutes at 350 F.
6. Mix chicken and spinach and serve on bowls.
7. Enjoy it!

Nutrition: Calories: 321, Fat: 9g, fruit 12g, Carbohydrates 22g, Protein: 17g.

Chapter 7. Desserts and Sweets Recipes

41.Peach Pie

(Ready in about 45 min | Servings 4 | Normal)

Ingredients:

One Pie dough

- 2 and 1/4 pounds of peaches pitted and sliced
- 2 tablespoons of cornstarch
- 1/2 cups of sugar
- 2 tablespoons of flour
- A shot of nutmeg, ground
- 1 tablespoon of dark rum
- 1 tablespoon of lemon juice
- 2 tablespoon of butter, molten

Directions:

1. Pull the pastry dough into a saucepan that suits the fryer and pressure well.
2. Balance the peaches in a bowl with the cornstarch, sugar, flour, nutmeg, rum lemon. Mix in milk, butter, and blend well.

3. Pour it into a pie pan, position the fryer and cook for 35 minutes 350° F.
4. Serve hot or cold.
5. Enjoy!

Nutrition: Calories: 231, Fat: 6g, Fiber: 7g, Carbohydrates 9g, Protein: 5g.

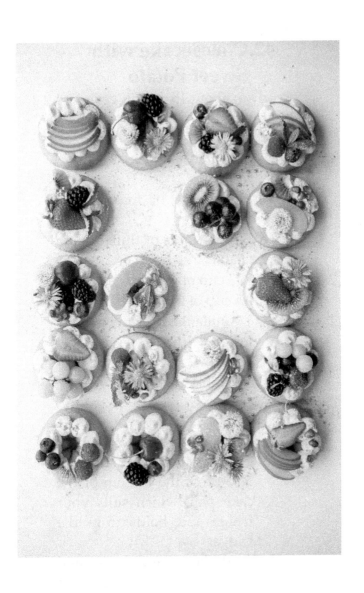

42. Cheesecake with Sweet Potato

(Ready in about 15 min | Servings 4 | Normal)

Ingredients:

- Four tablespoons of butter, molten
- Six ounces of mascarpone, mild
- Eight ounces of fluffy cream cheese
- 2/3 cup of graham
- 3⁄4 cup of milk
- 1 vanilla flavor extraction
- Puree with 2/3 cup sweet potato
- 1⁄4 tablespoons of ground cinnamon

Directions:

1. Comb butter and crumbled crackers in a pan, stir well and press the bottom of the cake pan, which suits your fridge and holds it in the fridge.
2. Blend the cream cheese and mascarpone in another container, sweet potato

puree, milk, espresso, and cinnamon and whisk very nicely.

3. Place over crust, placed in an AirFryer, cook at 300 °F. Hold in the fridge for four minutes, a few hours before serving, and enjoy!

Nutrition: Calories: 172, Fat: 4g, Fiber: 6g, Carbohydrates 8g, Protein: 3g.

43.Cookies with Brown Butter

(Ready in about 20 min | Servings 6 | Normal)

Ingredients:

- 1 and 1/2 cup of butter
- 2 cups of brown sugar
- Two whisked eggs
- Three cups of flour
- 2/3 cup of diced pecans
- Two vanilla tablespoons extract
- 1 teaspoon of baking soda
- 1/2 teaspoon of bake powder

Directions:

1. Heat a saucepan over a moderate flame with the butter, whisk till it melts, incorporate brown sugar and whisk until it decomposes.

2. In a cup, add pecan flour, vanilla extract, baking soda, baking, eggs, and flour, then mix well.

3. Apply brown butter, mix well and put a spoonful of this mixture on a lined sheet pan that perfectly fits your fryer.

4. Stir in the fryer and cook for 10 minutes at 340° F.
5. Cookies should be left to cool off and serve.
6. Enjoy!

Nutrition: Calories: 144, Fat: 5g, Fiber: 6g, Carbohydrates 19g, Protein: 2g

44.Bar Cashew

(Ready in about 25 min | Servings 6 | Normal)

Ingredients:
- 1/3 cup of honey
- 1⁄4 cup of almond meal
- 1 tablespoon of almond butter
- 1 and 1⁄2 cups of cashews
- 4 dates, sliced
- 3⁄4 cup of crushed coconut
- 1 spoonful of chia seeds

Directions:
1. Comb honey and almond butter in a cup, then mix well.
2. Insert cashews, coconut, chia seeds, and dates, and mix well again.

3. Place this on a rimmed baking sheet that works well with your AirFryer and press.
4. Stir in the fryer and cook for fifteen min at 300° Fahrenheit.
5. Leave the mixture to cool, cut to medium bars, and serve.
6. Enjoy it!

Nutrition: Calories: 121, Fat: 4g, Fiber: 7g, Carbohydrates 5g, Protein: 6g.

45. Tasty Orange Cookies

(Ready in about 22 min | Servings 8 | Normal)

Ingredients:

- 2 cups of flour
- 1 teaspoon of baking powder
- ½ cup of butter, soft
- ¾ cup of sugar
- 1 egg, whisked
- 1 teaspoon of vanilla extract
- 1 tablespoon of orange zest, grated

For the filling:

- 4 ounces of cream cheese, soft
- ½ cup of butter
- 2 cups of powdered sugar

Directions:

1. In a bowl, mix cream cheese with ½ cup butter and 2 cups powdered sugar, stir well using your mixer and leave aside for now.

2. In another bowl, mix flour with baking powder.

3. In a third bowl, mix ½ cup butter with ¾ cup sugar, egg,

vanilla extract, and orange zest and whisk well.

4. Combine flour with the orange mix, stir well and scoop one tablespoon of the mix on a lined baking sheet that fits your AirFryer.

5. Repeat with the rest of the orange batter, introduce in the fryer, and cook at 340° F for 12 minutes.

6. Leave cookies to cool down, spread cream filling on half of the top with the other cookies, and serve.

7. Enjoy!

Nutrition: Calories: 124, Fat: 5g, Fiber: 6g, Carbs: 8g, Protein: 4g.

46.Currant and Plum Tart

(Ready in about 1hr 5 min | Servings 6 | Difficult)

Ingredients:

For crumbling:

- 1/4 cup of almond flour
- One and a half cup of millet flour
- 1 cup of brown rice flour
- 1/2 cup of sugar cane
- 10 tablespoons of butter, mild
- Three tablespoons of milk

Filling for:

- 1 lb. of small, pitted, and halved plums
- 1 cup of white currant
- 2 tablespoons of cornstarch
- Three spoonfuls of sugar
- 1/2 teaspoon of strawberry extract
- 1/2 teaspoon of ground cinnamon
- 1/4 teaspoon of ground ginger
- 1 teaspoon of lime juice

Directions:

1. Mix the brown rice flour in a dish with 1/2 cup butter, millet meal, and almond flour, butter, and milk, then mix until you have a dough-like layer.
2. Put aside 1/4 of the dough, press the remaining dough into a tart pan to match. Fry the air and keep in the refrigerator for 30 minutes.
3. Meanwhile, blend the plums and currants in a cup, 3 tablespoons of sugar, cornstarch, vanilla extract, cinnamon, lime juice, and ginger, then mix well.
4. Pour over tart crust, crumble over reserved bread, put in your freeze air, and simmer for 35 minutes at 350° Fahrenheit.
5. Leave the tart to cool, cut, and slice.
6. Enjoy!

Nutrition: Calories: 200, Fat: 5g, Fiber: 4g, Carbohydrates 8g, Protein: 6g.

47.Plum Bars

(Ready in about 26 min | Servings 8 | Normal)

Ingredients:

- 2 cups of dry plums
- 6 tablespoons of water
- 2 cups of rolling oats
- 1 cup of brown sugar
- 1/2 teaspoon of baking soda
- 1 teaspoon of cinnamon powder
- 2 tablespoon of butter, melted
- 1 whisked egg
- Cooking spray

Directions:

1. Comb the plums with water in your mixing bowl and mix before you have a sticky stretch.
2. Mash oats and cinnamon in a tub, baking soda, sugar, egg, and butter, and whisk very strong.
3. Place half the oats in a baking saucepan, which matches your sprayed AirFryer, comb the plums with the frying oil,

and finish with the remaining half of the oats. Shake it up.

4. Stir in your AirFryer and cook for 16 minutes at 350° F.
5. Set the mixture aside to cool down, break into medium bars, and serve.
6. Enjoy it!

Nutrition: Calories: 111, Fat: 5g, Fiber: 6g, Carbohydrates 12g, Protein: 6g.

48.Sweet Squares

(Ready in about 40 min | Servings 6 | Normal)

Ingredients:

- 1 cup of flour
- Butter: 1/2 cup, mild
- 1 cup of sugar
- One and a half cup of powdered sugar
- Two spoons of lemon, rubbed
- Two tablespoons of lemon juice
- Two whisked eggs
- 1/2 teaspoon of powder

Directions:

1. Mix the flour with the ground sugar and butter in a tub, mix well, press the bottom of the saucepan that suits your fryer, put in the fryer, and bake for fourteen minutes at 350° Fahrenheit.

2. Comb sugar with lemon juice, lemon peel, eggs, and baking in another cup. Stir with the mixer, then sprinkle over the baked crust.

3. Bake for 15 minutes, allow to cool, cut into medium squares, and cool served.
4. Enjoy!

Nutrition: Calories: 100, Fat:s 4g, Fiber: 1g, Carbohydrates 12g, Protein: 1g.

Chapter 8. Lunch Recipes

49. AirFryer Chicken Fried Rice

(Ready in about 25min | Servings 2 | Easy)

Ingredients:
- 3 cups (325g) of rice cold
- 1 cup (130g) of chicken leftover and cubed
- 5 tbsp of tamari soy sauce or regular if not gluten-free
- 1.5 cup of frozen veggies (I used sweet corn and peas)
- 2 green onions (spring onions), sliced
- 1 tsp of sesame oil
- 1 tsp of vegetable oil
- 1 tbsp of chili sauce optional
- Salt to the taste

Directions:
1. The AirFryer is preheated to 350F/180C.
2. Combine all of the ingredients in a large tub.

3. Then switch to a non-stick pan which fits within the basket of the AirFryer.
4. Cook for 20 minutes before cooking, stirring the rice mixture a few times.

Nutrition: 6 Calories: 420kcal.

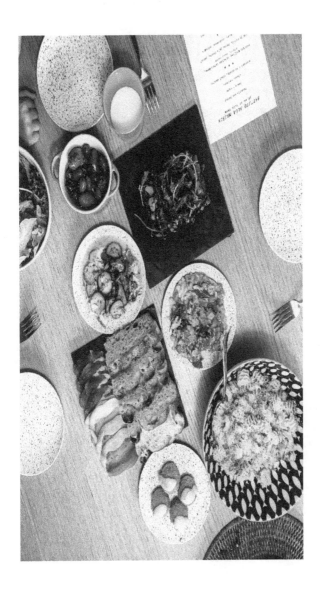

117

50. AirFryer fried Rice

(Ready in about 40 min | Servings 2 | Easy)

Ingredients:

- 300g of chicken tenderloins
- 4 rashers rindless bacon
- 450g of microwave long-grain rice
- 2 tablespoons of oyster sauce
- 2 tablespoons of light soy sauce
- 1 teaspoon of sesame oil
- 3 tsp finely grated fresh ginger
- 2 eggs, lightly whisked
- 120g (3/4 cup) of frozen peas
- 2 green shallots, sliced
- 1 long fresh red chili, thinly sliced
- Oyster sauce, to drizzle

Directions:

1. Preheat the fryer to 180C. Place the bacon and chicken onto the AirFryer shelf. Cook for eight minutes or until finished. Switch to a pan, and set aside slightly to cool.

Break the bacon into the chicken and chop.
2. Using the fingers meanwhile to break the rice grains in the box. Rice microwave for 1 minute. Switch to a 20 cm oval, ovenproof dish or cake pan with high edge. Stir in the oyster sauce, soy sauce, sesame oil, ginger, and water for 2 tbsp. Stir to blend.
3. Place the platter or saucepan in the AirFryer. Cook for about 5 minutes, or until the rice is fluffy. Drop the potato, peas, chicken, and bacon half cooked. Cook for 3 minutes or until the egg is overcooked. Add half of the shallot and sauté with salt and white pepper.
4. Serve with chili brushed, remaining shallot, remaining pork, and extra oyster sauce.

Nutrition: Calories: 400 kcal.

Conclusion

Air fryers are basically a small, turbo-powered convection oven for your kitchen countertop. It rapidly circulates hot air through the food to cook it quickly.

While the oil-less fryer has a removable basket like a regular fryer, instead of putting the food in hot oil, the food in the basket is cooked by the heat of the air circulating around it.

You can make anything you want! They allow you to cook practically anything: French fries that are usually crispy on the outside and fluffy on the inside; you can also make fried chicken, little fingers, nuggets, all frozen foods, fish, sausages, and even vegetables.